I0696279

Table of Contents

Understanding Heart Health

The Importance of a Healthy Heart

The heart is a vital organ that plays a crucial role in sustaining our overall health and well-being. It acts as a powerful pump, continuously circulating oxygen-rich blood to every part of the body. A healthy heart ensures that all organs and tissues receive the necessary nutrients and oxygen they need to function optimally. Understanding the importance of maintaining a healthy heart is key to preventing heart disease and living a long and fulfilling life.

Our heart works tirelessly, beating approximately 100,000 times a day. With each beat, it pumps blood through a network of blood vessels called the cardiovascular system. This intricate system supplies oxygen and nutrients to the body's cells and removes waste products. The heart's ability to perform this vital function efficiently is directly linked to our overall health and longevity.

Common Heart Conditions

Despite the heart's remarkable resilience, it is susceptible to various conditions that can impair its function and lead to serious health issues. Some common heart conditions include:

a) Coronary Artery Disease (CAD): This condition occurs when the arteries that supply blood to the heart become narrow or blocked due to the buildup of plaque. Reduced blood flow to the heart can cause chest pain (angina) and may lead to a heart attack if a complete blockage occurs.

b) Heart Attack: Also known as a myocardial infarction, a heart attack happens when blood flow to a part of the heart muscle is blocked, typically due to a blood clot. The lack of blood flow can cause damage or death to the affected heart tissue, resulting in severe chest pain, shortness of breath, and potentially fatal consequences.

c) Arrhythmias: Arrhythmias are irregular heart rhythms that can range from harmless to life-threatening. They occur when the electrical signals that regulate the heartbeat become disrupted, causing the heart to beat too fast, too slow, or irregularly.

d) Heart Failure: Heart failure is a chronic condition that happens when the heart cannot pump enough blood to meet the body's needs. It can result from various factors, including weakened heart muscle, high blood pressure, or previous heart attacks. Symptoms may include fatigue, fluid retention, and shortness of breath.

Risk Factors for Heart Disease

Understanding the risk factors associated with heart disease is crucial for prevention and early intervention. While some factors, such as age and family history, cannot be changed, there are several modifiable risk factors that individuals can address to reduce their risk of developing heart disease:

a) High Blood Pressure: Elevated blood pressure puts added strain on the heart and blood vessels, increasing the risk of heart disease and stroke. Lifestyle modifications and medication can help manage and control blood pressure.

b) High Cholesterol: An unhealthy balance of cholesterol in the blood, particularly high levels of LDL cholesterol (often referred to as "bad" cholesterol), can lead to the formation of plaque in the arteries. Adopting a heart-healthy diet and, if necessary, taking medications can help manage cholesterol levels.

c) Smoking: Smoking damages blood vessels, reduces oxygen supply to the heart, and increases the risk of heart disease. Quitting smoking is one of the most significant steps one can take to improve heart health.

d) Diabetes: Individuals with diabetes are at a higher risk of developing heart disease. Managing blood sugar levels through medication, a balanced diet, and regular exercise is essential for reducing this risk.

e) Obesity: Excess body weight, particularly abdominal obesity, increases the likelihood of developing heart disease. Adopting a healthy eating plan, engaging in regular physical activity, and achieving and maintaining a healthy weight can significantly reduce the risk.

f) Sedentary Lifestyle: Physical inactivity is a significant risk factor for heart disease. Engaging in regular exercise and reducing sedentary behaviors can enhance cardiovascular fitness and promote heart health.

Role of Nutrition in Heart Health

Proper nutrition is a cornerstone of maintaining a healthy heart and preventing heart disease. The food we eat directly impacts various risk factors associated with heart health, including blood pressure, cholesterol levels, blood sugar control, and body weight. Understanding the role of nutrition and making informed dietary choices can significantly improve heart health.

a) Healthy Fats: Consuming the right types of fats is crucial for heart health. Unsaturated fats, found in foods such as avocados, nuts, seeds, and olive oil, can help lower LDL cholesterol levels. On the other hand, saturated and trans fats, found in red meat, full-fat dairy products, and processed foods, should be limited as they can raise cholesterol levels.

b) Fiber: A high-fiber diet, particularly soluble fiber, can help lower LDL cholesterol levels and reduce the risk of heart disease. Including fruits, vegetables, whole grains, and legumes in the diet can provide an excellent source of dietary fiber.

c) Fruits and Vegetables: These plant-based foods are rich in antioxidants, vitamins, minerals, and dietary fiber. They promote heart health by reducing inflammation, improving blood pressure, and supporting overall cardiovascular function.

d) Sodium: High sodium intake is associated with increased blood pressure and an elevated risk of heart disease. Reducing sodium intake by limiting processed and packaged foods, and flavoring meals with herbs and spices instead of salt, can help maintain healthy blood pressure levels.

e) Omega-3 Fatty Acids: These essential fats, found in fatty fish (e.g., salmon, mackerel, sardines), walnuts, chia seeds, and flaxseeds, have been shown to have numerous heart-protective benefits. They can help reduce inflammation, lower triglyceride levels, and support overall heart health.

f) Plant Sterols: Plant sterols, naturally occurring compounds found in fruits, vegetables, and whole grains, can help lower LDL cholesterol levels. Consuming foods fortified with plant sterols or incorporating natural sources into the diet can have a positive impact on heart health.

g) Limiting Added Sugars and Refined Carbohydrates: A diet high in added sugars and refined carbohydrates has been linked to obesity, diabetes, and heart disease. Reducing consumption of sugary drinks, sweets, and refined grain products can lower the risk of heart disease.

Incorporating these heart-healthy nutritional principles into a well-balanced diet, along with regular physical activity, not only supports heart health but also contributes to overall wellness. It is important to consult with healthcare professionals and registered dietitians for personalized guidance and recommendations based on individual health conditions and needs.

By understanding the importance of a healthy heart, recognizing common heart conditions, identifying risk factors, and embracing the role of nutrition in heart health, individuals can take proactive steps toward maintaining a strong and vibrant heart, reducing the risk of heart disease, and enjoying a long and fulfilling life.

Part I: Foundation of a Heart-Healthy Diet

Building Blocks of a Heart-Healthy Diet

Eating a heart-healthy diet forms the foundation for promoting cardiovascular health and reducing the risk of heart disease. A well-balanced diet should consist of the right proportions of macronutrients (fats, carbohydrates, and proteins), an array of essential micronutrients (vitamins and minerals), an adequate intake of dietary fiber, mindful sodium and salt intake, and proper hydration. Let's delve into each of these building blocks to understand their role in supporting heart health.

2.1 Macronutrients: Fats, Carbohydrates, and Proteins

Macronutrients are the primary sources of energy for our bodies. It's important to choose the right types and quantities to maintain a heart-healthy diet.

a) Fats: Healthy fats play a crucial role in heart health. Monounsaturated and polyunsaturated fats, such as those found in avocados, nuts, seeds, and olive oil, can help reduce LDL cholesterol levels and lower the risk of heart disease. It's important to limit saturated and trans fats, found in red meat, full-fat dairy products, and processed foods, as they can increase LDL cholesterol and contribute to heart disease.

b) Carbohydrates: Carbohydrates provide energy for our bodies. Choosing complex carbohydrates, such as whole grains, legumes, fruits, and vegetables, is recommended for a heart-healthy diet. These sources provide fiber, vitamins, and minerals while minimizing added sugars and refined carbohydrates, which can raise the risk of heart disease.

c) Proteins: Including lean sources of protein, such as poultry, fish, legumes, and nuts, is important for a heart-healthy diet. These foods provide essential amino acids, vitamins, and minerals while being lower in saturated fats compared to red meat. It's crucial to balance protein intake with other macronutrients to maintain a well-rounded diet.

2.2 Micronutrients: Vitamins and Minerals

Micronutrients are vital for maintaining overall health, including heart health. Here are some key micronutrients and their role in supporting heart health:

a) Vitamins: B vitamins, including folate, B6, and B12, play a crucial role in maintaining heart health. They help reduce homocysteine levels, a compound associated with an increased risk of heart disease. Additionally, vitamins C and E, as antioxidants, help protect against oxidative stress and reduce inflammation, both of which are linked to heart disease.

b) Minerals: Minerals such as potassium, magnesium, and calcium are essential for heart health. Potassium helps regulate blood pressure, magnesium supports proper muscle and nerve function, and calcium contributes to heart muscle contraction. Including a variety of fruits, vegetables, whole grains, and dairy products can provide an adequate intake of these minerals.

Dietary Fiber

Dietary fiber is a type of carbohydrate that our bodies cannot fully digest. It plays a crucial role in maintaining heart health. There are two types of dietary fiber:

a) Soluble Fiber: Found in foods such as oats, barley, legumes, and fruits, soluble fiber forms a gel-like substance in the digestive system, helping to lower LDL cholesterol levels. It also promotes a feeling of fullness, which can aid in weight management.

b) Insoluble Fiber: Found in whole grains, nuts, seeds, and vegetables, insoluble fiber adds bulk to the stool and promotes regular bowel movements. It aids in maintaining a healthy digestive system and may help reduce the risk of developing certain types of cancers.

Including a variety of fiber-rich foods in the diet can help regulate blood cholesterol levels, maintain healthy blood sugar levels, promote satiety, and support overall heart health.

Sodium and Salt Intake

Sodium is an essential mineral required for various bodily functions. However, excessive sodium intake can raise blood pressure, increasing the risk of heart disease. It's important to be mindful of sodium consumption and monitor salt intake. Here are some tips to manage sodium intake:

a) Read Food Labels: Pay attention to the sodium content listed on food labels and choose lower-sodium options whenever possible. Opt for fresh, whole foods instead of processed and packaged foods, as they tend to be higher in sodium.

b) Limit Salt Usage: Be mindful of the amount of salt used in cooking and at the table. Experiment with herbs, spices, and other flavorings to enhance the taste of meals without relying heavily on salt.

c) Choose Low-Sodium Alternatives: When purchasing canned goods, choose low-sodium or no-salt-added options. Rinse canned vegetables and beans to reduce their sodium content.

By reducing sodium intake, one can help maintain healthy blood pressure levels and support heart health.

Importance of Hydration

Proper hydration is essential for overall health, including heart health. Staying adequately hydrated helps maintain blood volume, allowing the heart to pump blood more effectively. Here are some key points regarding hydration:

a) Water as the Best Beverage: Water should be the primary choice for hydration. It is calorie-free, does not contain added sugars or artificial sweeteners, and is readily available. Aim to drink enough water throughout the day to stay properly hydrated.

b) Limit Sugary Drinks: Sugary beverages, such as soda, fruit juices, and energy drinks, can contribute to weight gain, increase the risk of developing heart disease, and affect blood sugar levels. It's important to limit consumption of these beverages and opt for healthier alternatives like infused water, herbal tea, or unsweetened beverages.

c) Hydration and Physical Activity: During physical activity, proper hydration is crucial for maintaining optimal performance and preventing dehydration. Drink water before, during, and after exercise to replace fluids lost through sweating.

d) Individual Hydration Needs: It's important to remember that individual hydration needs may vary depending on factors such as climate, activity level, and overall health. Pay attention to your body's signals of thirst and aim to drink water consistently throughout the day.

Maintaining proper hydration supports overall cardiovascular health, promotes healthy blood circulation, and helps the heart function optimally.

By understanding and implementing the building blocks of a heart-healthy diet, including appropriate macronutrient choices, essential micronutrients, dietary fiber, mindful sodium and salt intake, and proper hydration, individuals can support their cardiovascular health, reduce the risk of heart disease, and enhance their overall well-being.

Understanding Heart Health: Key Nutrients for Heart Health

3.1 Omega-3 Fatty Acids

Omega-3 fatty acids are a group of essential fats that are crucial for heart health. They are polyunsaturated fats that cannot be produced by the body, so they must be obtained through the diet. There are three main types of omega-3 fatty acids: alpha-linolenic acid (ALA), eicosapentaenoic acid (EPA), and docosahexaenoic acid (DHA).

a) ALA: Found in plant-based sources such as flaxseeds, chia seeds, and walnuts, ALA is converted in the body into EPA and DHA, although the conversion is limited. Nonetheless, ALA still offers cardiovascular benefits, including reducing inflammation and blood clotting.

b) EPA and DHA: These omega-3 fatty acids are predominantly found in fatty fish like salmon, mackerel, and sardines. EPA and DHA are directly associated with various heart-protective effects. They can help lower triglyceride levels, reduce blood pressure, decrease inflammation, improve arterial function, and prevent the formation of blood clots.

Including omega-3-rich foods in the diet or considering supplementation, particularly for individuals who do not consume fish, can provide significant benefits for heart health.

3.2 Antioxidants

Antioxidants are compounds that protect the body's cells from damage caused by harmful molecules called free radicals. Free radicals can contribute to oxidative stress and inflammation, both of which are associated with the development of heart disease. Including antioxidant-rich foods in the diet can help counteract these effects and promote heart health.

a) Vitamin C: Found in citrus fruits, strawberries, bell peppers, and leafy green vegetables, vitamin C is a potent antioxidant that helps protect against oxidative stress and inflammation. It also plays a role in collagen synthesis, which is important for maintaining the health of blood vessels.

b) Vitamin E: Nuts, seeds, vegetable oils, and leafy green vegetables are excellent sources of vitamin E. This fat-soluble vitamin acts as an antioxidant and helps prevent the oxidation of LDL cholesterol, reducing the risk of plaque formation in the arteries.

c) Flavonoids: Flavonoids are a diverse group of antioxidants found in fruits, vegetables, tea, and dark chocolate. They have been associated with several heart-protective benefits, including reducing inflammation, improving blood pressure, and enhancing arterial function.

By incorporating a wide variety of colorful fruits, vegetables, nuts, seeds, and other antioxidant-rich foods into the diet, individuals can support their heart health and reduce the risk of heart disease.

3.3 Potassium

Potassium is a mineral that plays a crucial role in maintaining heart health. It helps regulate blood pressure by counteracting the effects of sodium and relaxing blood vessel walls. Adequate potassium intake has been associated with a lower risk of developing high blood pressure and reducing the risk of stroke.

Good dietary sources of potassium include bananas, oranges, avocados, leafy green vegetables, potatoes, and legumes. By including these foods in the diet, individuals can increase their potassium intake and support heart health.

It's important to note that individuals with certain health conditions, such as kidney disease, may need to limit their potassium intake. Consulting with a healthcare professional or registered dietitian can provide personalized guidance based on individual needs.

3.4 Magnesium

Magnesium is an essential mineral involved in various processes in the body, including heart function and maintaining healthy blood pressure levels. It helps relax blood vessels, supports proper muscle function, and contributes to the regulation of heart rhythm.

Magnesium-rich foods include leafy green vegetables, whole grains, nuts, seeds, legumes, and dark chocolate. Consuming a balanced diet that incorporates these foods can help ensure an adequate intake of magnesium and promote heart health.

3.5 Calcium

Calcium is well-known for its role in supporting bone health, but it also plays a vital role in heart health. It helps regulate muscle contractions, including the heart muscle, and supports proper nerve function. Adequate calcium intake has been associated with a lower risk of developing high blood pressure and reducing the risk of cardiovascular disease.

Good dietary sources of calcium include dairy products, such as milk, cheese, and yogurt, as well as fortified plant-based milk alternatives, leafy green vegetables, tofu, and almonds. Consuming a variety of calcium-rich foods can help meet the body's calcium needs and support heart health.

It's important to note that excessive calcium intake from supplements may increase the risk of heart disease, particularly in individuals who already have or are at risk for cardiovascular problems. It is generally recommended to obtain calcium through dietary sources rather than supplements, and consulting with a healthcare professional or registered dietitian can provide personalized guidance.

By incorporating omega-3 fatty acids, antioxidants, potassium, magnesium, and calcium through a well-balanced diet, individuals can nourish their hearts and support cardiovascular health. Remember that a diverse and colorful array of foods is key to obtaining these essential nutrients.

Understanding Cholesterol and Heart Health

Cholesterol plays a crucial role in the body, but an imbalance in cholesterol levels can significantly impact heart health. In this section, we will explore the different types of cholesterol, understand the importance of managing cholesterol levels, and discover the impact of dietary choices on cholesterol.

4.1 Differentiating between Good and Bad Cholesterol

Cholesterol is a waxy substance produced by the liver and also obtained through dietary sources. It is essential for the production of hormones, vitamin D synthesis, and the formation of cell membranes. However, cholesterol can be categorized into two types based on its transport in the bloodstream:

a) Low-Density Lipoprotein (LDL) Cholesterol: LDL cholesterol is often referred to as "bad" cholesterol. It carries cholesterol from the liver to the body's cells. When LDL cholesterol levels are too high, it can build up in the walls of arteries, forming plaque. This can narrow the arteries and restrict blood flow, increasing the risk of heart disease, heart attacks, and strokes.

b) High-Density Lipoprotein (HDL) Cholesterol: HDL cholesterol is commonly known as "good" cholesterol. It acts as a scavenger, picking up excess cholesterol from the bloodstream and tissues and returning it to the liver for processing and excretion. Higher levels of HDL cholesterol are associated with a lower risk of heart disease.

Maintaining a healthy balance between LDL and HDL cholesterol is vital for heart health. High levels of LDL cholesterol and low levels of HDL cholesterol can increase the risk of developing heart disease.

4.2 Managing Cholesterol Levels

Managing cholesterol levels is an essential aspect of maintaining heart health. Elevated LDL cholesterol levels are a major risk factor for the development of heart disease. Here are some strategies for managing cholesterol levels:

a) Regular Cholesterol Screening: Regular cholesterol screenings can help identify imbalances in cholesterol levels. It is recommended to have a complete lipid profile, including measurements of total cholesterol, LDL cholesterol, HDL cholesterol, and triglycerides, at least once every four to six years for adults.

Individuals with known risk factors or those diagnosed with high cholesterol may need more frequent screenings.

b) Lifestyle Modifications: Making lifestyle changes is often the first line of defense in managing cholesterol levels. These modifications include adopting a heart-healthy diet, engaging in regular physical activity, maintaining a healthy weight, quitting smoking, and managing stress levels. Lifestyle modifications can help lower LDL cholesterol levels, raise HDL cholesterol levels, and reduce the risk of heart disease.

c) Medications: In some cases, lifestyle modifications may not be sufficient to manage cholesterol levels. In such instances, healthcare professionals may prescribe medications, such as statins, to help lower LDL cholesterol levels. These medications work by inhibiting the production of cholesterol in the liver.

4.3 Impact of Dietary Choices on Cholesterol

Dietary choices play a significant role in managing cholesterol levels. Certain foods can raise LDL cholesterol levels, while others can help lower them. Here are some key dietary considerations for maintaining healthy cholesterol levels:

a) Saturated Fats: Saturated fats, found primarily in animal-based foods such as fatty meats, full-fat dairy products, and tropical oils like coconut oil, can raise LDL cholesterol levels. It is recommended to limit the intake of saturated fats and choose healthier alternatives like lean meats, low-fat dairy products, and plant-based oils such as olive oil.

b) Trans Fats: Trans fats, often found in processed and commercially baked goods, increase LDL cholesterol levels and decrease HDL cholesterol levels. It is important to read food labels and avoid products that list "partially hydrogenated oils" in the ingredients. Opt for healthier fats like monounsaturated fats (found in avocados, nuts, and olive oil) and polyunsaturated fats (found in fatty fish, seeds, and nuts) instead.

c) Dietary Fiber: Including soluble fiber in the diet can help lower LDL cholesterol levels. Foods rich in soluble fiber include oats, barley, legumes, fruits, and vegetables. Aim to incorporate these fiber-rich foods into your meals and snacks to support healthy cholesterol levels.

d) Plant Sterols and Stanols: Plant sterols and stanols are naturally occurring compounds found in certain plant-based foods. They have been shown to reduce LDL cholesterol levels. Foods fortified with plant sterols or stanols, such as margarine spreads or specific brands of orange juice, can be incorporated into the diet for added benefits.

e) Omega-3 Fatty Acids: Omega-3 fatty acids, particularly those found in fatty fish like salmon, mackerel, and sardines, have been shown to have heart-protective effects. They can help lower triglyceride levels and may have a modest impact on raising HDL cholesterol levels. Including omega-3-rich foods or considering supplementation can be beneficial for managing cholesterol levels.

f) Alcohol Consumption: While moderate alcohol consumption has been associated with a modest increase in HDL cholesterol levels, excessive alcohol intake can raise triglyceride levels and contribute to other health problems. It is recommended to consume alcohol in moderation, which means up to one drink per day for women and up to two drinks per day for men.

By making mindful dietary choices, individuals can positively impact their cholesterol levels and support heart health. It's important to remember that dietary changes should be made in conjunction with overall lifestyle modifications and under the guidance of healthcare professionals or registered dietitians.

Understanding the different types of cholesterol, managing cholesterol levels through lifestyle modifications and, if necessary, medications, and making informed dietary choices are vital steps toward maintaining a healthy heart and reducing the risk of heart disease.

DUKAN DIET AND COOKBOOK

From Katherine Jenkins and Jennifer Lopez to Pippa and Carole Middleton, Dukan Diet recipes have a well-known fan base. Probably the reason it was the best selling diet book in Britain, when it was first released in 2010.

A 'breakthrough' diet book by Dr Pierre Dukan, his low-fat eating, high-protein eating plan has been credited with quick weight loss for people that might otherwise find dieting difficult.

And now you can eat gourmet food and still lose weight! Diet guru Monica Grenfell gives us the lowdown...

Dr Pierre Dukan's high-protein diet has been a favourite with French women for 10 years' says Monica. 'You need discipline to follow it: the rule is no fruit, no treats, no alcohol and no carbs for as long as it takes to lose your excess weight.

Your reward will be the pounds rolling off. And now the new book with recipes by a Michelin-starred chef has made this a gourmet's diet, too.'

How does the Dukan Diet work?

Dr Dukan devised the weight-loss method around 4 phases: two for losing weight, and two for stabilising the weight you get down to, all using a list of 100 'permitted' foods from which you can eat as much as you want.

The 4 phases are called: Attack, Cruise, Consolidation and Stabilisation. In the first two, you are limited to the 100 foods permitted, which are used to make up tasty recipes.

Duken diet meal plan:

Phase 1: Attack

You start with 72 lean protein foods during Attack, including: steak, veal, liver, reduced fat ham, reduced fat bacon, cooked chicken or turkey slices, cod, sole, haddock, salmon, sardines, tuna, shellfish, virtually fat-free cottage cheese, virtually fat-free quark, fat-free yogurt, skimmed milk, eggs and tofu.

First 5 days

You kick-start your weight loss with five days of eating only protein on the Dukan Diet – from the 72 high-protein foods, plus 1-2tbsp milled oat bran a day for fibre.

In the first phase of the diet, you can eat high protein foods such as cheese, milk and yogurt

Breakfast

Coffee/tea with skimmed milk

Fat-free yogurt Dukan pancake

-Stir 1½tbsp oat bran with 1½tbsp non-fat fromage frais, 1 egg, sweetener or salt. Cook for 2 mins each side)

Serve with Dukan nutella

-Mix 1 egg yolk, 1tsp reduced-fat cocoa powder, 2tbsp sweetener and a little water)

Lunch

Egg, smoked salmon and Dukan mayonnaise

-Combine 1 egg yolk and 1tbsp Dijon mustard. Season and add 1tbsp chopped parsley or chives.

Gradually stir in 3tbsp virtually fat-free fromage frais or quark

Dinner

Rosemary meatballs

-Mix 1 diced onion; 750g minced beef; 2 crushed garlic cloves; 1 egg, lightly beaten; 1tbsp Worcestershire sauce; 2tbsp Chinese plum sauce; 2tbsp rosemary, 1-2tbsp mint or basil, all finely chopped; salt and black pepper. Shape into balls the size of a walnut. Cook in batches over a medium heat, for 5 mins or until golden. Drain away fat before serving.

Lemon Mousse

-Soak 2 gelatine leaves in a bowl of cold water for a few mins. Add 2tbsp sweetener, the grated zest of ½ lemon and 50g fromage frais to 1 egg yolk. Whisk, then warm in a pan for 2 mins. Remove and stir in the drained and squeezed gelatine. Whisk 200g fromage frais and fold into the lemon cream. Beat 1 egg white until stiff and fold in. Refrigerate until set.

Phase 2: Cruise

Then add the 28 vegetables during Cruise, including: artichoke, fennel, onions, asparagus, French beans, aubergine, leek, beetroot, courgette, mushrooms, broccoli, cabbage, pepper, carrots, pumpkin, celery, tomatoes, salad leaves and swede. Follow until you reach your goal weight

In the Cruise phase of the Dukan Diet, keep eating all the foods you were allowed on Attack, and add the 28 vegetables to your diet. The idea is to alternate days of protein only with protein and vegetable days. You stay on Cruise until you have lost all the weight you want to shed.

In the second phase, you can add 28 vegetables to your diet, such as beans, leek and broccoli

Protein and Vegetable Day

Breakfast

As Phase 1 (Attack)

Lunch

Quick gazpacho

-Poach 4 tomatoes in boiling water for 30 secs, then peel and deseed them. Grill 1 red pepper and 1 green pepper for 10-15 mins until charred. Place in a plastic bag to cool, before peeling away the skin and seeds and cutting into chunks. Blend the tomatoes and peppers with 2 cucumbers (peeled, deseeded and chopped) and some mint in a blender. Season and serve chilled.

Dinner

Chicken with mushrooms

-Thinly slice 600g button mushrooms. Sprinkle over a few drops of lemon juice and put them in a non-stick casserole dish. Season, cover and cook over a gentle heat until all their water has evaporated. Drain and put to one side. Brown 1 chopped onion in a casserole dish in a little water. Add 800g chicken breasts, cut into cubes; 2 chopped tomatoes; the mushrooms; 2 chopped garlic cloves; 250ml low-salt chicken stock; salt and pepper. Cover and cook over a gentle heat for 20 mins.

Phase 3: Consolidation – One night off a week

Once you have reached your goal weight, the Dukan Diet moves on from the 100 natural foods to allow bread, pasta and fruit. You have one evening a week when you can eat whatever you like. Thursday remains a protein-only day to help you keep to your goal weight.

Calculate how long you need to stay on Consolidation by multiplying every pound you lost by five, e.g., 7lb x 5 = 35 days

n phase 3, you're allowed to eat bread and pasta again. Hurrah!

Eat

• As much protein and vegetables (together) each day as you want.

- 1 fruit a day – but not high sugar bananas, grapes, cherries or dried fruits. Watermelon, an apple or papaya are best.

- 2 slices wholemeal bread per day, with reduced-fat butter.

- One serving (40g) of hard cheese per day – avoid blue cheese, soft cheese or goat's cheese.

- One serving per week of 'starchy foods' such as pasta or rice in the first half of your Consolidation phase, increasing to two portions per week in the second half.

- Pasta and tomato sauce. You may also have chickpeas, lentils, couscous, polenta and potatoes.

- Relax a little and enjoy one night out or 'special' meal in the first half of your Consolidation phase, increasing to two in the second half. In this meal you really can eat anything you like!

- Make Thursday your protein-only day.

Phase 4: Stabilisation – Staying slim

Congratulations, you've done it! So now you can relax and return to eating and drinking normally, but make sure that every Thursday remains a protein-only day to help you keep the weight off for good.

Day 1

Breakfast: scrambled eggs with smoked salmon (serves 1)

Whisk 2 eggs in a bowl. Add a splash of skim milk. Add as much chopped smoked salmon as you like. Microwave on high for 1 minute. Stir. Microwave for another 30 seconds and serve.

Lunch : ham rolls (serves 4)

175g extra-lean ham, finely chopped

225g fat-free quark*

Finely chopped chives and marjoram, to taste

4 shallots, finely chopped

Tabasco, to taste

Mix all ingredients and roll into small balls.

Dinner: Vietnamese beef (serves 2)

400g sirloin steak, cut into 1cm cubes

2 tbs soy sauce

1 tbs oyster sauce

1 big piece ginger, grated

3 drops vegetable oil

4 garlic cloves, crushed

Coriander leaves, to serve

Combine beef, sauces, ginger and a little black pepper. Marinate for at least 30 minutes. Brown garlic in a pan (oiled and wiped with kitchen paper). Add beef and stir over high heat for 10-15 seconds for medium-rare. Top with coriander.

Day 2

Breakfast: yoghurt (serves 1)

200g fat-free yoghurt sprinkled with oat bran, 1 drop of vanilla essence and sweetener.

Lunch: oat bran pancake (serves 1)

1½ tbs oat bran

1½ tbs fat-free quark

Dried herbs, optional

175g flaked tuna, smoked salmon, ham or chicken

2 eggs, separated

Oil, for cooking

Stir oat bran into quark with herbs, a pinch of salt and pepper, fish, meat or chicken and egg yolks. Beat eggwhites until stiff peaks form, then fold into oat bran mixture. Pour into a non-stick pan that has been oiled and wiped with kitchen paper and a few drops of oil. Cook for 2-3 minutes each side.

Dinner: baked fish with herbs (serves 4)

800g white fish fillets

300g fat-free fromage frais

4 eggs

5 tbs chopped herbs

3 drops vegetable oil

Preheat oven to 220ºC. Season fish fillets and wrap in greaseproof paper. Bake for 10 minutes. Reduce heat to 180ºC. Remove fish from oven. Put cooked fillets into a blender with fromage frais, eggs and herbs and blend well. Pour mixture into a baking dish (oiled and wiped with kitchen paper). Place dish into a bigger dish. Half fill bigger dish with cold water. Bake for 45 minutes or until cooked through.

Dessert: lemon cheesecake

2 eggs

4 tbsp fromage frais

4 tbsp quark

200g cottage cheese

300g fat-free cream cheese

2 tbsp cornflour

8 tbsp sweetener

grated lemon zest

Heat oven to 160ºC. Mix ingredients except egg whites and cornflour and beat until smooth and thick. In another bowl, beat the egg whites until stiff, then add the cornflour.Fold this mixture into the first bowl. in a dish, bake for 40 minutes or until risen and golden brown. Cool, then serve garnished with grated lemon zest.

Day 3

Breakfast: oat bran porridge (serves 1)

Combine 2 tbs of oat bran and a little wheat bran (optional) with skim milk and sweetener. Microwave for 2 minutes.

Lunch: rosemary beef burgers (serves 3)

750g minced beef

1 onion, chopped

2 garlic cloves, crushed

2 tbs plum sauce

1 tbs Worcestershire sauce

2 tbs finely chopped rosemary

1-2 tbs finely chopped mint or basil

1 egg, lightly beaten

Salad to serve, optional

Combine all ingredients, season with salt and pepper to taste and shape into patties. Grill until golden brown on both sides and cooked through. Drain on paper towel.

Dinner: fishcake (serves 1)

3 eggs, separated

6 tbs fat-free quark

1 tbs cornflour

1 garlic clove, crushed

Chopped herbs, to taste

1 white fish fillet, chopped

3 crabsticks, thinly sliced

Beat eggwhites until stiff. Add other ingredients and bake in a lined tin at 180ºC for 45 minutes.

Dessert: chocolate coffee meringues

3 egg whites

2 tsp cocoa powder

6 tbsp sweetener

2 tsp very strong coffee

Preheat the oven to 150ºC. Beat the egg whites until very stiff. Add the cocoa to the sweetener, then sprinkle this over the egg whites. Add the coffee and continue beating for about 30 seconds. Spoon into small mounds on a baking tray and bake for 25 to 30 minutes.

Day 4

Breakfast: oat bran muffins (serves 4)

4 eggs, separated

8 tbs oat bran

4 tbs fromage frais

1/2 tsp sweetener

Lemon zest or cinnamon

Heat oven to 180ºC. Beat eggwhites until stiff. Mix other ingredients. Fold in eggwhites. Pour into cases. Bake for 20-30 minutes.

Lunch: prawn and egg salad (serves 2)

1 tsp olive oil

4 tsp cider vinegar

600g lettuce

A few sprigs tarragon

200g prawns, cooked and shelled

4 eggs

Make a vinaigrette with oil and vinegar and some salt and pepper. Mix lettuce, tarragon leaves and prawns in a bowl.

Soft-boil eggs for 5-6 minutes. Shell carefully as yolks will still be runny. Serve eggs, while still very hot, on top of dressed lettuce and prawns.

Dinner: salmon escalopes and mustard dill sauce (serves 4)

4 thick (about 200g each)

pieces salmon

2 shallots, chopped

1 tbs mild mustard

6 tsp fat-free fromage frais

Finely chopped dill, to taste

Steamed asparagus,optional

Put salmon in the freezer for a few minutes so you can cut it into thin (about 50g) slices. Gently fry slices in a non-stick pan for 1 minute each side. Set aside and keep warm. Brown shallots. Reduce heat. Add mustard and fromage frais. Simmer for 5 minutes. Return salmon to pan. Add dill. Season. Cook until heated through. Serve with asparagus.

Dessert: chocolate pannacotta (serves 1)

2 gelatine leaves

2 egg yolks

1 tbsp of cocoa powder

1 tbsp protein powder

100ml skimmed milk

5 tbsp fat-free fromage frais

Place the gelatine in a bowl of cold water to soften. In another bowl, combine the egg yolks, cocoa powder and protein powder, set aside. Bring the milk to the boil in a small saucepan, gently pour over the egg mixture and stir to combine.

Squeeze out any excess water from the gelatine and drop into the hot mixture, then stir until fully dissolved. Allow to cool, then add the fromage frais.

Day 5

Breakfast: muesli and skim milk (serves 2)

6 tbs oat bran

1 egg

1 tbs liquid sweetener

Almond essence

Preheat oven to 160ºC. Mix all ingredients and spread on tray lined with baking paper. Bake for 30 minutes. Crumble when cool. Store in an air-tight container.

Lunch: salmon pancakes (serves 2)

300g fat-free fromage frais

60g fat-free quark

1 small jar salmon roe

4 slices smoked salmon

2 oat bran pancakes

(see Day 2 lunch recipe)

Mix fromage frais, quark and roe in a bowl. Season. Divide mixture among pancakes. Top with salmon.

Dinner: chicken kebabs (serves 4)

1 onion, peeled

1 garlic clove, peeled

20g ginger, grated

2 tbs lemon juice

100g fat-free plain yoghurt

1/2 tbs ground coriander

1/2 tbs ground cumin

1 tsp garam masala

2 tbs finely chopped coriander

800g chicken breasts, cut into 2cm chunks

Fat-free tzatziki, to serve

Purée onion and garlic in a blender. Stir in ginger, lemon juice, yoghurt, spices and coriander. Mix chicken and marinade in a bowl. Refrigerate for 2 hours. Heat a grill on high.

Thread chicken on skewers. Cook for 8-10 minutes. Serve with fat-free tzatziki.

Dessert: orange yogurt cake

3 eggs

150g fat-free natural yogurt

½ tsp artificial sweetener

1tsp orange extract

4 tbsp cornflour

2 tsp yeast

3 drops of vegetable oil

Preheat the oven to 180ºC. Beat eggs with yogurt, then add sweetener, orange extract, corn flour and yeast. Pour into a cake tin (oiled and lined with kitchen paper) and bake for 45 minutes.

Snacks

• Low-fat yogurt sprinkled with oat bran a drop of vanilla flavouring and sweetener

• Sugar-free jelly

• Hard boiled egg

• Cold chicken

• Carrot sticks with low-fat cheese or yoghurt

Tips on Dukan Diet

- Tip 1: Stock up on protein. "For best results on the Attack phase, make sure you are well-stocked with plenty of proteins—especially fresh proteins," says Gloger. "Prepare your proteins in bulk: meatballs, burger patties, filets, ground meat, steaks, hard-boiled eggs etc. The more lean protein and fresh water you have on hand, the better your results."

- Tip 2: Avoid sodium traps. "You can season the proteins in any way, but avoid table salt and use Himalayan or Celtic sea salt instead. The sodium content in prepackaged proteins (chicken/tuna in a can, deli meat, mock crab, etc.) can be quite high, so use fresh protein instead."

- Tip 3: Drink a lot. "Try to have eight glasses of water a day. Herbal teas are an optimal choice and count toward your water intake—great for cold winter days!"

- Tip 4: Oat bran is your friend. "Make sure to have your oat bran! [The only carb allowed on the diet.] In the Attack Phase, 1.5 tablespoons are allowed per day. Try to have your oat bran during the times of day that you are hungriest or experience the most cravings. You can have your oat bran as a hot cereal, pancake, muffin, in your yogurt, or as breading for your proteins."

• Tip 5: Expect to feel a little off. "It's normal—don't quit! Your hunger will disappear after the third day due to the increased release of ketones in the body, which are powerful natural hunger suppressants. Headaches or dizziness are due to sugar withdrawal. The symptoms should pass in three or four days once you wean your body off this metabolism killer." Of course, it's best to take any negative symptoms seriously, so don't hesitate to contact your doctor if you ever are concerned about how you feel on any diet plan.

Simone's Typical Meal Plan (in the Cruise Phase)

- ___Breakfast:2 organic pasture-raised eggs and oat bran hot cereal with cinnamon, black organic coffee

- Snack: Vital Choice wild salmon burger or tofu/tempeh

- Lunch: Chop't salad with romaine, kale, carrots, beets, cucumbers, broccoli, and chicken tossed with red wine vinegar

- Snack: Dukan Turkey Jerky

- Dinner: Fish or chicken with vegetables and shirataki noodles or a big salad with a can of wild salmon or tuna

MondayDay 1

Breakfast

- Warm drink

- Low fat cottage cheese

- 2 slices of grilled chicken breast

Lunch

- Vietnamese Beef

- Low fat yoghurt

Tea

- Cinnamon Oat Bran Pancake

Dinner

- Garlic Tiger Prawns

- Garlic chicken slices

TuesdayDay 2

Breakfast

- Warm drink

- Omelette

- Several ham slices (less than 5% fat)

Lunch

- Trout with herbs

- Prawns

Tea

- Tea or coffee without sugar

- Vanilla Oat Bran Porridge

Dinner

- Hard boiled eggs

- Dukan Mayo

WednesdayDay 3

Breakfast

- Warm drink

- Low fat cream cheese

- Turkey ham slices

Lunch

- Grilled chicken breast

- Muesli ice-cream

Tea

- Pink Cheesecake Cupcakes

Dinner

- Oat bran chicken nuggets

- Kogel Mogel

ThursdayDay 4

Breakfast

- Warm drink

- Scrambled eggs

- Low fat cream cheese

Lunch

- Chicken Curry

Tea

- Tea or coffee, no sugar

- Oat bran muffins

Dinner

- Salmon Soup

FridayDay 5

Breakfast

- Warm drink

- Low fat yoghurt with oat bran

Lunch

- Steamed fish with herbs

- Low fat cottage cheese

Tea

- Surimi sticks

Dinner

- Peppered beef steak

SaturdayDay 6

Breakfast

- Warm drink

- Mint & Curry Omelette

Lunch

- Grilled turkey breast steaks

- Ham slices

Tea

- Oat bran cookies

- Diet soda

Dinner

- Baked Turkey Meatballs

SundayDay 7

Breakfast

- Warm drink

- Soft Boiled Eggs with Meaty Crisps

Lunch

- Smoked Salmon Appetizers

- Oat bran pancake

Tea

- Tea or coffee without sugar

Dinner

- Roast Chicken (without skin)

What to drink on the Dukan Diet

Drinking plenty is a very important part of the Dukan diet, especially during protein days. The suggested 2-3 litres of liquids per day can seem like a daunting task when you start the diet, however you will quickly learn that it's not only managable, but can help you enjoy your meals and avoid cravings.

One thing we should get out of the way first is that liquids does not mean just water. You are encouraged to drink with every meal any of the following:

water

bottled, sparkling, or tap

tea

no sugar, but you can use sweeteners or skimmed milk; herbal tea is allowed too

coffee

no sugar, but you can use sweeteners or skimmed milk

diet sodas

diet pepsi, coke zero, or any other sugar-free drink

Here's a day of typical meals during Dukan's first three phases. "The Dukan Diet" guide provides meal plans for the "Attack" and "Cruise" phases. Although technically all-you-can-eat, portions have been applied to calculate nutritional analyses. Your diet may differ from what appears below.

While "The Dukan Diet" guide offers no menu for the Consolidation phase, U.S. News assembled one based on its guidelines. Here, too, your menu may differ from what appears below.

Finally, because the "Permanent Stabilization" phase is shaped almost entirely by you, no sample meal plan is provided.

Attack Phase

Breakfast

8 fluid ounces coffee with artificial sweetener of your choice

8 ounces nonfat yogurt

1 Dukan oat-bran galette (pancake)*

Snack (if hungry)

4 ounces nonfat cottage cheese

Lunch

Hard-boiled egg with herb mayonnaise*

5 ounces barbecue steak*

8 ounces nonfat yogurt

Snack (if hungry)

4 ounces nonfat yogurt

Dinner

1 pound shrimp sauteed in herbs

8 ounces tandoori chicken cutlets

Dukan custard*

Cruise Phase

Breakfast

8 fluid ounces coffee with artificial sweetener of your choice

8 ounces nonfat yogurt

1 oat-bran galette (pancake)*

Snack (if hungry)

4 ounces nonfat cottage cheese

Lunch

Lettuce salad with vinaigrette*

Cauliflower gratin*

Custard*

Snack (if hungry)

4 ounces nonfat yogurt

Dinner

Cucumbers, served hot or cold*

8 ounces chicken Marengo*

Vanilla creme*

Consolidation Phase

Breakfast

8 ounces coffee with artificial sweetener of your choice

8 ounces nonfat yogurt

1 oat-bran galette (pancake)*

2 slices whole-grain bread with 2 teaspoons light butter

Snack (if hungry)

4 ounces nonfat cottage cheese

1 apple

Lunch

Lettuce salad with vinaigrette*

Cauliflower gratin*

Custard*

Snack (if hungry)

4 ounces nonfat yogurt

1 1/2 ounces cheddar cheese

Dinner

Cucumbers, served hot or cold*

8 ounces chicken Marengo*

8 ounces cooked quinoa

Vanilla creme

100 Foods Allowed on the Dukan Diet

"You don't lose weight when you're hungry"

During his research, Pierre Dukan identified 100 allowed foods that contain the essential nutrients for our bodies that have tremendous benefits and are rich in protein, low in carbohydrates and fat. You can eat as much as you want from the Dukan Diet food list during the four phases of the Dukan Diet.

68 Pure Proteins: Starting on the Attack phase

 Lean meat

Beef tenderloin, Filet mignon – Buffalo – Extra-lean ham – Extra-lean Kosher beef hot dogs – Lean center-cut pork chops - Lean slices of roast beef - Pork tenderloin, pork loin roast – Reduced-fat bacon, soy bacon- Steak: flank, sirloin, London broil– Veal chops – Veal scaloppini - Venison

Poultry

Chicken – Chicken liver – Cornish hen – Fat-free turkey and chicken sausages – Low fat deli slices of chicken or turkey – Ostrich steak - Quail – Turkey - Wild duck

Fish

Arctic char – Catfish – Cod – Flounder – Grouper – Haddock – Halibut and smoked halibut – Herring – Mackerel – Mahi Mahi – Monkfish – Orange roughy – Perch – Red snapper – Salmon or mmoked salmon – Sardines, fresh or canned in water – Sea bass – Shark - Sole – Surimi – Swordfish – Tilapia – Trout – Tuna, fresh or canned in water

Shellfish

Clams – Crab – Crawfish, crayfish – Lobster – Mussels – Octopus – Oysters – Scallops – Shrimp - Squid

Vegetarian Proteins

Seitan – Soy foods and veggie burgers – Tempeh - Tofu

Fat-free dairy products

Fat-free cottage cheese, Fat-free cream cheese, Fat-free milk, Fat-free plain Greek style yogurt, Fat-free ricotta, Fat-free sour cream

Eggs

Chicken – Quail – Duck

And Sugar-free gelatin

Artichoke - Asparagus – Bean sprouts - Beet - Broccoli - Brussels sprouts - Cabbage - Carrot - Cauliflower - Celery - Cucumber - Eggplant - Endive - Fennel - Green beans – Kale – Lettuce, arugula, radicchio – Mushrooms – Okra – Onions, leeks, shallots – Palm Hearts - Peppers – Pumpkin - Radishes – Rhubarb - Spaghetti squash - Squash - Spinach – Tomato – Turnip – Watercress – Zucchini

Although the Dukan Diet book has been a bestseller for years in France, it's been rapidly gaining popularity since Kate Middleton reportedly started the diet in order to lose weight for her upcoming royal nuptials to Prince William. Other celebs like model Giselle Bundchen and Jennifer Lopez are also said to have tried the diet to help them shed their post-baby pounds. But should you be following in the footsteps of these high-profile celebs? We're breaking down the basics (and the risks) of this hot diet.

Overview

Poor carbs! They can never catch a break. The new version of Atkins has arrived. Followers of the Dukan diet indulge in unlimited lean protein, but must eliminate carbohydrates (including fruits and veggies) completely, at least during the first phase. French physician Pierre Dukan created the diet over a decade ago as a means to treats obese individuals, but the slew of celebrity followers and their weight-loss brought it into the spotlight. As such, the Dukan diet fad has hit the U.K. by storm, and its gaining ground in the U.S.

The Plan

Just like Atkins, this plan has four phases, with lean protein being the main focus. During each phase, oat bran, tons of water and a 20-minute daily walk is required. It's suggested that dieters take a multivitamin with minerals. Here is a breakdown of each of them:

• Phase 1- The "Attack" Phase: Unlimited amounts of lean protein, 1.5 tablespoons of oat bran and 1.5 liters of water per day. Choose from a selection of 72 lean or low-fat meats, fish, poultry, pork, soy, eggs, and non-fat dairy (not including lamb.)

• Phase 2- The "Cruise" Phase: In addition to the low-fat proteins and oat bran (increased to 2 tablespoons), say hello to 32 vegetable options every other day. Some veggies that aren't allowed: sweet carrots and peas, corn and starchy potatoes.

• Phase 3- Consolidation: This less-restrictive phase allows unlimited protein (including lamb) and veggies every other day. New allowable foods include one piece of low-sugar fruit, 1 portion of hard cheese, and 2 slices of whole grain bread each day. A few servings of starchy foods and celebration meals are also allowed each week. During this phase, you'll also choose one day each week (preferably Thursday or the same day each week) to eat only protein.

• Phase 4- Stabilization: The final stage of this plan is maintenance. During this phase you can eat whatever you like as long as you follow a few simple rules: one day per week follow phase 1, and eat 3 tablespoons oat bran and walk for 20 minutes each day.

The Costs

Dieters be warned! Expect to be hungry for the first 3 days on this diet, but Dr. Dukan claims hunger will disappear on day 4. In addition to hunger, other side effects of this diet include constipation, dry mouth, fatigue and bad breathe.

Weight loss on this diet is inevitable since there is a significant drop in the amount of calories you'll eat. However, the rate of weight loss is too quick, which can promote gallstones and muscle loss. Additionally, since most food groups are eliminated, you won't be getting in all your nutrients (including vitamins and minerals), which are needed to maintain a healthy body.

The Good

• Protein selection is from lean protein sources like fish, poultry, eggs and soy.

• No weighing foods or calorie counting

The Not-So-Good

• It's a very restrictive diet where most healthy food groups are eliminated.

• The rate of rate loss is too rapid and unsafe.

• Side effects of constipation, bad breath, dry mouth and fatigue.

• Healthy eating habits are not learned on this plan.

• High protein diets can lead to kidney failure, dehydrates and overconsumption of unhealthy fats (like saturated) and cholesterol, which have been linked to heart disease.

• How much protein can someone realistically eat?!?

• Tough to eat while traveling or on the go.

The Bottom Line: This restrictive diet is unhealthy and impractical. Just like Atkins came and went, so will the Dukan Diet. A well-balanced diet with all of the food groups is the way to go.

Raspberry Cheesecake

Ingredients for the sponge (tray with 18-20 cm diameter):

-2 egg whites

- 1 egg yolk

- 1 tsp konjac flour (or 1 tbsp corn starch)

- 2 tbsp oat bran

- 2 tbsp sweetener

- vanilla flavouring

Cheese-layer ingredients:

-500 fat free cream cheese (ricotta, Philadelphia))

- 150g fat free greek yogurt

- 1 egg

Cinnamon & Caramel Cheesecake

Ingredients:

-500 g Philadelphia cheese, or other lox-fat soft cheese

- 150 g greek yogurt or low fat soured cream

- 2 eggs

- 4-5 tbsp sweetener

-2 tbsp corn starch (only from Cruise phase)

Pain Doux (French Sweet Bread)

Ingredients:

-4 eggs

- 4 tbsp oat bran

- 6 tbsp skimmed milk powder

- 4-5 tbsp powdered sweetener

- 1 tsp vanilla essence

- 1 tbsp baking powder

Baked chicken with cherry tomatoes and peppers

Ingredients:

-4-5 boneless chicken thighs

- 2 peppers

- 6-8 cherry tomatoes

- 1-2 cloves of garlic

- 1 tbsp olive oil

-2 tsp italian herbs

- salt, pepper

- 250 ml water or chicken broth

How to prepare:

1. Preheat oven to 350 degrees F (175 degrees C)

2.Place the chicken thighs in a pan or oven

Baked Chicken with Vegetables

Ingredients:

-2-4 Chicken drumsticks

- 1 red pepper

- 1 onion

- 1 zucchini

- 2 cloves of garlic

-3-4 Cherry tomatoes

- 1 tbsp olive oil

- ½ tbsp sweet paprika

- ½ tbsp garlic powder

- Salt and pepper

- 1 tbsp oregano

How to prepare:

1. Preheat oven to 350 degrees F (175 degrees C).

Baked Chicken with Vegetables

Ingredients:

-2-4 Chicken drumsticks

- 1 red pepper

- 1 onion

- 1 zucchini

- 2 cloves of garlic

-3-4 Cherry tomatoes

- 1 tbsp olive oil

- ½ tbsp sweet paprika

- ½ tbsp garlic powder

- Salt and pepper

- 1 tbsp oregano

How to prepare:

1. Preheat oven to 350 degrees F (175 degrees C).

2.Cut the vegetables into larger cubes and put them in the tray

3.Mix olive oil with sweet paprika, garlic powder, salt, pepper and oregano.

4. Brush the chicken drumsticks with this olive mix and put them over vegetables in the tray

5. Add water to the pot (about a cup)

6. Cover with aluminum foil or a lid and put into the oven

7. Cook in the oven about 40-45 minutes, then remove foil or lid and cook another 10-15 minutes

Enjoy your dukan meal!

Proscuitto Wrapped Asparagus with Egg

Dukan Phases: Cruise Phase, Consolidation Phase, Stabilization Phase

Servings: 4

Serving Size: 1 bundle with 1 egg

Nutritional Info: 93 calories, 5g of fat, 4.8g of carbohydrates, 2.4g of fiber, 8.9g of protein

Ingredients

1 pound fresh asparagus

4 pieces proscuitto, ham, or bacon

Salt and pepper

4 eggs

Instructions

1. Heat oven to 400 F. Trim the asparagus and season with salt and pepper.

2. Divide the asparagus into four servings. Wrap each with a piece of proscuitto (ham or bacon).

3. Place the wrapped bundles onto baking sheet and bake for 20 minutes.

4. During the last 5 minutes of cooking, cook 4 eggs over easy in a skillet to serve on top.

Spicy Stuffed Cucumbers

Dukan Phases: Cruise Phase, Consolidation Phase, Stabilization Phase

Servings: 4

Serving Size: 5 cucumber slices

Nutritional Info: 54 calories, .3g of fat, 7.8g of carbohydrates, 1.1g of fiber, 6.7g of protein

Ingredients

2 cucumbers

3/4 cup nonfat Greek Yogurt

1 minced garlic clove

1/2 tsp. paprika

2 tsp. fresh chopped dill

1/2 tsp. chili powder or couple splashes hot sauce

Optional: Up to 1/2 cup crab, salmon, tuna, or canned chicken breast

Instructions

1. Mix together the yogurt, garlic, paprika, dill, and chili powder. Let refrigerate for at least 45 minutes.

2. Cut cucumbers into rounds and scoop out most of the inside using a spoon.

2. Fill each cucumber with yogurt mixture and tip with chili powder or paprika.

Miso Soup

Dukan Phases: Attack Phase, Cruise Phase, Consolidation Phase, Stabilization Phase

Servings: 2

Serving Size: 1 cup

Nutritional Info: 68 calories, 2g of fat, 2g of carbohydrates, 1g of fiber, 8g of protein

Ingredients

2 cups chicken or vegetable broth

1 tbsp. white miso paste

1 tsp dashi granules

2 tbsp. dried seaweed

2 scallions, chopped

Instructions

1. Bring the broth to a boil.

2. Whisk in the miso paste and dashi granules.

3. Simmer for 5 minutes. Stir in the green onion and dried seaweed.

Chive Pancakes

Dukan Phases: Attack Phase, Cruise Phase, Consolidation Phase, Stabilization Phase

Servings: 1

Serving Size: 2 pancakes

Nutritional Info: 124 calories, 5.1g of fat, 10g (from oat bran) of carbohydrates, .7g of fiber, 10g of protein

Ingredients

2 tbsp. of oat bran

1 tbsp. of nonfat powdered milk

1 egg

1/4 tsp. baking soda

Salt and pepper

1 tbsp. chives

Instructions

1. Whisk together the oat bran, powdered milk, egg, baking soda, salt, and pepper.

2. Fold in the chives.

3. Cook in a nonstick skillet coated with cooking spray. Cook for 3-4 minutes per side.

Dukan Lime Granita

Dukan Phases: Attack Phase, Cruise Phase, Consolidation Phase, Stabilization Phase

Servings: 4

Serving Size: 1/4 recipe

Nutritional Info: 8 calories, 0g of fat, 2.1g of carbohydrates, 0g of fiber, 0g of protein

Ingredients

1/2 cup lime juice

1 tsp. lime zest

1 cup water

Stevia to taste (start with 1 tablespoon and move up)

Instructions

1. Combine the lime juice, lime zest, water, and Stevia in a bowl. Stir together well. Taste and adjust sweetness to your liking by adding more Stevia.

2. Pour the mixture into a large baking dish. It shouldn't be more than one inch deep.

3. Place in the freezer. After one hour, remove and scrap with 1-2 forks to break up the ice.

4. Place back in the freezer and continuing scraping every 30-40 minutes until everything has turned to ice flakes.

Dukan Spicy Mussels

Dukan Phases: Attack Phase, Cruise Phase, Consolidation Phase, Stabilization Phase

Servings: 4

Serving Size: 1/4 recipe

Nutritional Info: 263 calories, 6.8g of fat, 1g of carbohydrates, 1g of fiber, 20g of protein

Ingredients

2 shallots, sliced

1 inch ginger, sliced

4 garlic cloves, sliced

2 Thai chiles (or Serranos)

1 cup water

2 tbsp. fish sauce (or soy sauce)

2 lbs, cleaned mussels

Instructions

1. Add everything except the mussels to a large pot and bring to a summer. Let simmer for 5 minutes.

2. Add the mussels and cover immediately.

3. Steam for 5-7 minutes until mussels open up.

Dukan Diet Shrimp Fajitas

Dukan Phases: Cruise Phase, Consolidation Phase, Stabilization Phase, Veg and Protein

Servings: 2

Serving Size: 1/4 recipe

Nutritional Information: 282.9 calories, 4.2 g of fat, 12 g of carbohydrates, 2.5 g of fiber, 47.6 g of protein

Ingredients

2 tsp. ancho chile powder

2 tsp. salt

1 tsp. cumin

1 tsp. onion powder

1/2 tsp. garlic powder

4 tbsp. fresh lime juice

2 lbs. shrimp, shelled and deveined

1 green pepper, sliced

1 red pepper, sliced

1 onion, sliced thin

1 cup sugar snap peas

1 jalapeno, sliced thin

Instructions

Mix together all the spices to create your fajita seasoning.

Toss the shrimp in 4 tbsp. of the fajita seasoning and 2 tbsp. of lime juice. Let marinate for 10 minutes. Store the remaining fajita seasoning.

Heat a skillet over medium heat and spray with cooking spray. Add the shrimp and cook for about 2 minutes per side until just cooked. Remove and set aside.

Add the veggies and cook for 5-7 until softe. If needed add a couple of tablespoons of water to prevent sticking or burning.

Add the shrimp back to the pan. Serve with cauliflower rice or in lettuce wraps.

Dukan Garlic Clams

Dukan Phases: Attack Phase, Cruise Phase, Consolidation Phase, Stabilization Phase

Servings:4

Serving Size: 1/2 pound

Nutritional Info: varies based on shellfish used, around 290 calories

Ingredients

3/4 cup water

4 tbsp. lemon juice

1 onion, minced

3 garlic cloves, minced

3 garlic cloves, whole

1 tsp. dried thyme (1 tbsp. fresh)

1 lb. clams, cleaned

Salt and pepper to taste

Instructions

1. Heat a skillet with a cover or Dutch oven over medium heat. Spray with cooking spray and add the onion, garlic, and thyme and cook for 5 minutes.

2. Add the water, lemon juice, salt, pepper, and shellfish. Cover and cook for 6-9 minutes or until shells open up and fish is cooked through.

Dukan Slow Cooker Rotisserie Chicken

Dukan Phases: Attack Phase, Cruise Phase, Consolidation Phase, Stabilization Phase

Servings:4

Serving Size: 8 crackers

Nutritional Info: 62.2 calories, 3.9g of fat, 7.6g carbohydrates, 2.2g dietary fiber, 3.1g of protein

Ingredients

2 packets of rapid rise active yeast

1 cup warm water

1 cup of oat bran

1 tsp. olive oil

1/4 tsp. salt

Pepper

Instructions

1. Add the yeast to the warm water and let rest for 10 minutes until it bubbles.

2. Add the oat bran, olive oil, salt, and pepper and stir together until a sticky dough forms.

3. Form into a ball and cover with a towel. Let rise for at least one hour.

4. Preheat the oven to 430 degrees with a baking sheet inside.

5. Roll the dough out to form an 16 by 16 square. You can roll it out between two sheets of parchment paper to keep it from sticking. Cut into 32 crackers.

6. Remove the hot baking sheet and place a new piece of parchment on it. Lay out the crackers and bake for 10 minutes. Flip over and bake for 10 more minutes or until dry and crispy.

Dukan Slow Cooker Rotisserie Chicken

Dukan Phases: Attack Phase, Cruise Phase, Consolidation Phase, Stabilization Phase

Servings:varies

Serving Size: varies

Nutritional Info: varies per piece

Ingredients

1 3 lb. chicken, cleaned with fat removed

1 tsp. smoked paprika

1/2 tsp. salt

1/2 tsp. pepper

1/2 tsp. garlic powder

1/2 tsp. dried basil

1/2 tsp. dried oregano

1 lemon

Instructions

1. Make 3-5 aluminum balls and place in the bottom of the slow cooker.

2. Mix together all of the spices and add the juice of the lemon. Rub the spice rub all over the chicken.

3. Stuff the lemon into the chicken cavity and place on top of the aluminum foil balls or wrapped potatoes.

4. Cook on low for 8 hours.

Optional: For crispy skin, preheat the oven to 500 degrees and roast the chicken for 10 minutes before serving to crisp up the skin.

Dukan Baked Lemon Chicken Legs

Dukan Phases: Attack Phase, Cruise Phase, Consolidation Phase, Stabilization Phase

Servings: 4 servings

Serving Size: 1 chicken leg quarter

Nutritional Info: varies based on size and if you leave the skin on

Ingredients

☐ 4 chicken leg quarters, skin removed during Attack phase

☐ Juice of 2 lemons

☐ 2 tbsp. olive oil

1 tsp dried rosemary

☐ 1 tsp steak seasoning

☐ 4 cloves garlic, minced

☐ Salt and pepper

☐ 4-8 thin slices lemon.

Instructions

1. Preheat the oven to 325 degrees.

2. Stir together the lemon juice, olive oil, rosemary, steak seasoning, garlic, salt, and pepper. Toss the chicken in the marinade and let sit for 30 minutes.

3. Dump everything into a glass baking dish. Place the chicken skin side down. Roast for 45 minutes and flip the chicken over. Place the lemon slices on top of the skin.

4. Roast for another 45 minutes or until juice run clear and the internal temperature reaches 170.

Dukan Italian Flank Steak Pinwheels

Dukan Phases: Attack Phase, Cruise Phase, Consolidation Phase, Stabilization Phase

Servings: 4 servings

Serving Size: 1/4 recipe

Nutritional Info: 140 calories, 5.4g of fat, 0g carbohydrates, 0g dietary fiber, 21.6g of protein

Ingredients

☐ 1 tsp. olive oil

☐ 1 lb. 95% lean ground beef, chicken, or turkey

☐ 1 garlic clove, minced

☐ Salt and pepper

☐ 2 tsp. madras curry powder

Instructions

1. Heat the olive oil over medium high heat.

2. Add the garlic and beef and break into smaller pieces using the back of a spoon.

3. Cook until the meat is cooked through and no pink remains.

4. Add the curry powder, salt, and pepper. Taste and adjust seasoning if needed.

Dukan Italian Flank Steak Pinwheels

Dukan Phases: Cruise Phase, Consolidation Phase, Stabilization Phase

Servings: 4 servings

Serving Size: 1/4 recipe

Nutritional Info: 248.3 calories, 11.7g of fat, 5.4g carbohydrates, 1.3g dietary fiber, 29.9g of protein

Ingredients

☐ 1 lb. flank steak, trimmed of fat

☐ Salt and pepper

☐ 1 garlic clove

☐ 1.5 cups spinach, packed, chopped

☐ .5 cups basil, chopped

☐ 1/2 cup sundried tomatoes, packed in water, chopped

☐ 3/4 cup part skim mozzarella cheese

☐ 2 tsp. olive oil

Instructions

1. Pound the flank steak out until it is ¼ thick or butterfly it. *You can also ask the butcher to do this for you)

2. Season both sides of steak well with salt and pepper,

3. Rub one side of the steak with garlic clove.

4. Layer the spinach, basil, and sundried tomatoes evenly across the steak, leaving 1 inch around edges. Top with cheese.

5. Start at one edge and roll up tightly.

6. Secure using toothpicks or a kabob skewers. (If you use toothpicks soak them in water for 20 minutes prior to make sure they don't catch on fire.)

7. Brush the outside of the steak with oil.

8. Option 1: Cut the steak into 8 portions and grill or pan sear each for 3-4 minutes per side.

9. Option 2: Grill the entire rolled steak whole. It will take about 15-20 minutes for medium rare and you will need to flip it throughout to prevent burning. Let rest, tented in foil, for ten minutes before slicing and serving.

Dukan Sauteed Mini Mushroom Frittatas

Dukan Phases: Cruise Phase, Consolidation Phase, Stabilization Phase

Servings: 12 servings

Serving Size: 1 muffin

Nutritional Info: 80.1 calories, 4.7g of fat, 1.8g carbohydrates, .3g dietary fiber, 7.8g of protein

Ingredients

1 tbsp unsalted butter

1 medium yellow onion, sliced very thin

1/2 tsp finely chopped fresh thyme leaves

8 ounces cremini mushrooms, cleaned and sliced

4 oz reduced fat Swiss cheese

4 whole eggs

8 egg whites

2 tablespoons skim milk

.5 tsp Worcestershire

1 tsp salt

Salt and pepper

Instructions

1. Preheat the oven to 350.

2. Bring a saute pan to medium low heat and add the butter. Once melted, add the onions and cook for about 30-45 minutes until deep brown and caramelized. Stir when needed to prevent burning. Once finish stir in the thyme and season with salt and pepper to your liking.

3. Remove the onions from the pan and add the mushrooms. Cook for about ten minutes until softened and season with salt and pepper to your liking. There should be enough residual butter leftover so the mushrooms don't burn, but if needed add some cooking spray. Mix together with the onions when finished.

4. While the mushrooms are cooking, whisk together the eggs, egg whites, milk, salt, and Worcestershire. Stir in the cheese.

5. Spray your muffin tin with cooking spray. Divide the mushroom mixture between the 12 cups, saving 12 mushrooms slices if you want to place them on top. Then pour the egg mixture over. Add the mushroom slice if you would like them for the top. This is purely decorative.

6. Bake for about 15 minutes until cooked through. Let rest for 5-10 minutes before serving. Delicious warm or cold.

Dukan Sauteed Cocktail Shrimp

Dukan Phases: Attack Phase, Cruise Phase, Consolidation Phase, Stabilization Phase

Servings: 4 servings

Serving Size: 1/4 recipe

Nutritional Info: 130.1 calories,3.1 g of fat, 1 g of carbohydrates, 0 g of fiber 23 g of protein

Ingredients

1 tsp olive oil

1 pound jumbo shrimp, peeled and deveined

1 tbsp herbes de Provence

Salt and pepper

Instructions

1. In a skillet, heat the oil over medium-high heat.

2. Add the shrimp and herbes de Provence. Season with salt and pepper.

3. Cook until the shrimp are pink and cooked through. It should take about 2 minutes each side.

Dukan Slow Shrimp and Tofu Miso Soup

Dukan Phases: Attack Phase, Cruise Phase, Consolidation Phase, Stabilization Phase

Servings: 6 servings

Serving Size: 1.5 cups

Nutritional Info: 241 calories, 5 g of fat, o g of carbohydrates, .22 g of fiber 42.3 g of protein

Ingredients

- ☐ 6 cups vegetable broth (or chicken broth)

- ☐ 1/4 cup soy sauce

- ☐ 1 tablespoon ginger, peeled and minced

- ☐ 1/2 tsp Asian chili paste

- ☐ 5 tablespoons miso

- ☐ 2 lbs shrimp, peeled

- ☐ 1 cup tofu, cut into chunks

- ☐ 4 cups spinach, trimmed and chopped roughly or seaweed (do not use during Attack Phase)

- ☐ 1/2 cup green onion, sliced

Instructions

1. Add the broth, ginger, chili paste, and soy sauce to a large pot. Bring to a simmer over medium high heat.

2. In a small bowl whisk the miso with 1/2 cup hot broth.

3. Add the mixed miso into the pan.

4. Bring to a boil and add the shrimp, spinach, tofu, and green onions. Cook for about 5 minutes or until shrimp is cooked through.

Dukan Slow Cooker Shredded Beef

Dukan Phases: Attack Phase, Cruise Phase, Consolidation Phase, Stabilization Phase

Servings: 8 servings

Serving Size: 1 cup

Nutritional Info: 225 calories, 9.6 g of fat, o g of carbohydrates, 0 g of fiber 32 g of protein

Ingredients

2 1/2 pound beef roast, trimmed of all fat

Kosher salt

Freshly ground black pepper

1 cup beef broth

1/2 cup apple cider vinegar

2 tsp smoked paprika

1 tsp chili powder

1 tsp garlic powder

1 tsp onion powder

1 tsp cumin

1 tsp dried oregano

Instructions

1. Mix together all of the dry spices and rub them on the beef.

8. 2. Add the beef to the slow cooker with 1 cup of beef broth.

9. 3. Cook on low for 8 hours until the beef easily shreds with a fork.

Dukan Cauliflower Soup

Dukan Phases: Cruise Phase, Consolidation Phase, Stabilization Phase

Servings: 8 servings

Serving Size: 1 cup

Nutritional Info: 46.4 calories, 1.9 g of fat, 6.6 of carbohydrates, 2.9 g of fiber 2.2 g of protein

Ingredients

1 tsp olive oil

1 medium onion, sliced thin

1 large head fresh cauliflower

Salt, to taste

1 tsp fresh thyme

4 1/2 cups hot water, divided

Black pepper, to taste

Instructions

1. In a large pot, heat the olive oil over medium low heat. Cook for about 15 minutes until they soften up and become fragrant.

2. Add the cauliflower, salt and pepper, and 1 cup water. Bring the heat to medium and bring it to a simmer. Cover the pot and let everything cook for about 15 minutes until the cauliflower is fork tender.

3. Add the remaining water and thyme and continue to simmer for 20 minutes.

15. 4. Puree the soup using an immersion blender or regular blender. Let stand for 20 minutes so it thickens up.

Dukan Diet Broccoli Soup

Dukan Phases: Cruise Phase, Consolidation Phase, Stabilization Phase

Servings: 8

Serving Size: 1 cup

Nutritional Info: 61.6 calories, 3.5 g of fat, 3 g carbohydrates, 1.3 g dietary fiber, 5.8 g of protein

Ingredients

2.5 pounds broccoli, chopped

1 medium onion, chopped

2 garlic cloves, minced

1 1/2 tsp dry mustard powder

1/2 tsp Cayenne powder

1/4 tsp baking soda

4 cups chicken broth

3 oz sharp low fat cheddar, grated

1 1/2 oz parmesan, grated

Salt and pepper to taste

Instructions

1. Heat a large pot sprayed with cooking spray over medium heat add the broccoli, onion, garlic, mustard powder, cayenne, and about 1 tsp salt. Cook for about 5 minutes until the broccoli becomes fragrant.

2. Add 1 cup of chicken broth and the baking soda and bring to a simmer. Cook until the broccoli is soft and tender, about 20 minutes.

3. Add remaining broth broth and bring the soup to a simmer. Add the cheese and then blend using an immersion blender or carefully in a regular blender. Season with salt and pepper.

Dukan Diet Mushroom Omelet

Dukan Phases: Cruise Phase, Consolidation Phase, Stabilization Phase

Servings: 1

Serving Size: 1 omelet

Nutritional Info: 112 calories, 6.1 g of fat, 2.1 g carbohydrates, 0.4 g dietary fiber, 14.1 g of protein

Ingredients

Cooking spray

2 oz mushrooms, cleaned and sliced

1/2 tsp fresh thyme, minced

1 garlic clove, minced

1 egg and 2 egg whites

1 tbsp non-fat milk

2 tsp chopped parsley

1 tsp chopped chives

Salt and pepper to taste

2 tbsp fat free cheese

Instructions

1. Heat a non stick skillet over medium high heat. Add the mushrooms and cook for 3 minutes and

then add the thyme, garlic, salt, and pepper. Cook for 3 more minutes and set aside.

2. Whisk together the eggs, milk, salt, pepper, parsley, and chives.

3. Add the eggs to the non stick pan over medium heat. Let cook mostly through and the flip to the other side. Add the mushrooms and cheese and fold in half to serve.

Dukan Diet Turkey Burgers

Dukan Phases: Attack Phase, Cruise Phase, Consolidation Phase, Stabilization Phase

Servings: 4

Serving Size: 1 burger

Nutritional Info: 191.5 calories, 9.2 g of fat, 2.8 g carbohydrates, 0.8 g dietary fiber, 24.7 g of protein

Ingredients

1 pound lean ground turkey

1 egg and 1 egg white, lightly beaten

1 tsp teaspoon sea salt

2 tsp Old Bay seasoning

1 red bell pepper, minced (do not use during Attack phase)

1/4 cup onion, minced

2 tbsp parsley, minced

Instructions

1. Using your hands, combine all the ingredients until just mixed.

2. Cook burgers in a non-stick skillet for about 7 minutes on each side until completely cooked through.

Dukan Diet Deviled Eggs

Dukan Phases: Attack Phase, Cruise Phase, Consolidation Phase, Stabilization Phase

Servings: 24

Serving Size: 1 egg half

Nutritional Info: 37 calories, 1.7 g of fat, 1.3 g carbohydrates, 0 g dietary fiber, 3.8 g of protein

Ingredients

12 large eggs

1/2 cup plain fat-free Greek yogurt

1 tablespoon Dijon mustard

1 to 2 teaspoons hot pepper sauce

1/8 teaspoon salt

1/8 teaspoon paprika

1/8 teaspoon black pepper

2 tablespoons chopped green onions

Instructions

1. Add the egg to a large sauce pan and cover with water. Bring the water to a boil and then remove the heat. Cover and let stand for about 15 minutes and remove to let cool.

2. Once the eggs have cooled, peel them. Then slice in half and remove the yolks. Keep 6 yolks and throw away the remaining yolks or save for another recipe.

3. Combine the yogurt, mustard, hot sauce, salt, paprika, pepper, and egg yolks in a bowl. Mix until well blended using a hand mixer.

4. Spoon about 1 tablespoon of the mix into each egg half and garnish with green onions or chives.

Dukan Diet Eggplant Rollatini

Dukan Phases: Cruise Phase, Consolidation Phase, Stabilization Phase

Servings: 4

Serving Size: 1/4 recipe

Nutritional Info: 147 calories, .2 g of fat, 30 g carbohydrates, 3.7 g dietary fiber, 28.8 g of protein

Ingredients

1 large eggplant

16 oz fat free ricotta cheese

4 oz fat free mozzarella cheese

1/2 can diced tomatoes with Italian seasoning

2 tbsp Italian seasoning

Salt and pepper to taste

Instructions

1. Lay eggplant on a baking sheet sprayed with a non-stick spray; place into a 350°F oven for 10 minutes and then turn eggplant. Cook other side till lightly browned. Cooking times will vary with each oven.

2. In a large mixing bowl combine the ricotta, mozzarella, 1/2 the diced tomatoes, Italian seasoning, salt, and pepper.

Dukan Diet Grilled Citrus Salmon

Dukan Phases: Attack Phase, Cruise Phase, Consolidation Phase, Stabilization Phase

Servings: 4

Serving Size: 6 oz salmon

Nutritional Info: 313 calories, 13 g of fat, 1 g carbohydrates, 0 g dietary fiber, 43.2 g of protein

Ingredients

Juice from 1 orange

Juice from 2 lemons

Juice from 2 limes

1/2 cup cilantro

1/2 teaspoon sugar

1/2 cup chopped onion

1 inch ginger, grated

4 6 oz salmon fillets

Directions

1. Mix together all of the ingredients, except the salmon, in a bowl and add to a ziploc bag.

2. Add the salmon and marinate for one hour.

3. Remove salmon and pat dry with a paper towel. Season with salt and pepper. Grill on medium high heat for about 4 minutes per side or until cooked to your liking. Serve with extra citrus.

3. Add about 2 tbsp of the cheese mixture onto each piece of eggplant and roll. Place in a baking dish and cover with additional diced tomatoes.

Bake for 10-15 minutes until the cheese begins to bubble on the sides.

www.ingramcontent.com/pod-product-compliance
Lightning Source LLC
Chambersburg PA
CBHW070806260726